THIS JOURNAL BELONGS TO

______________________________

SHE

BELIEVED

SHE COULD

SO SHE

DID

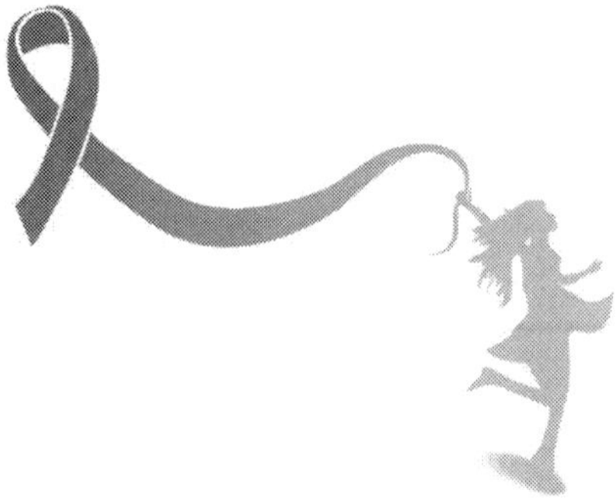

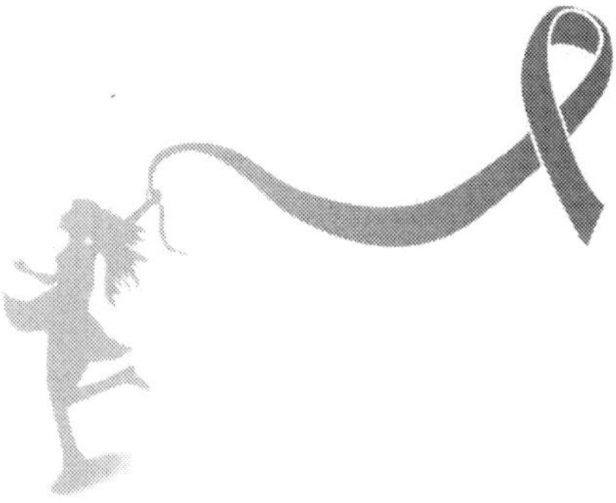

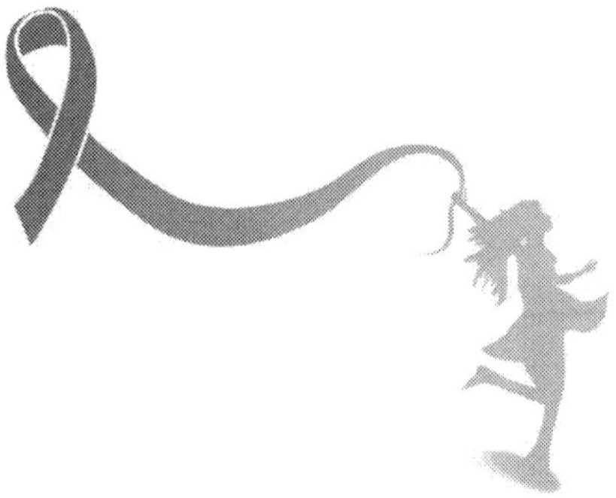

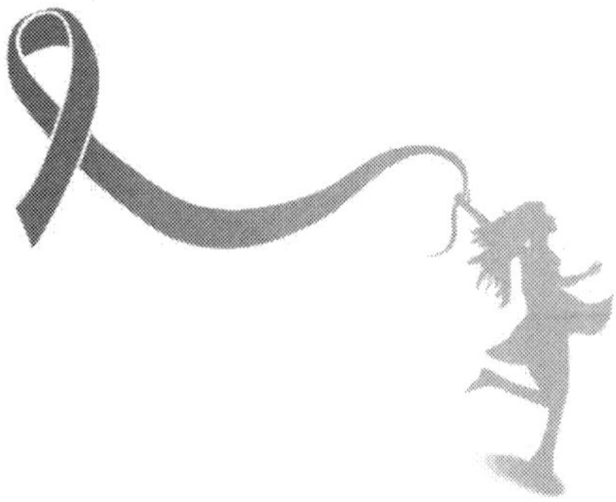

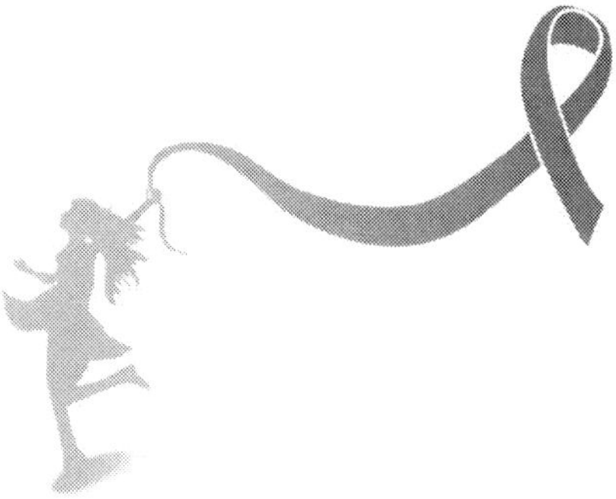

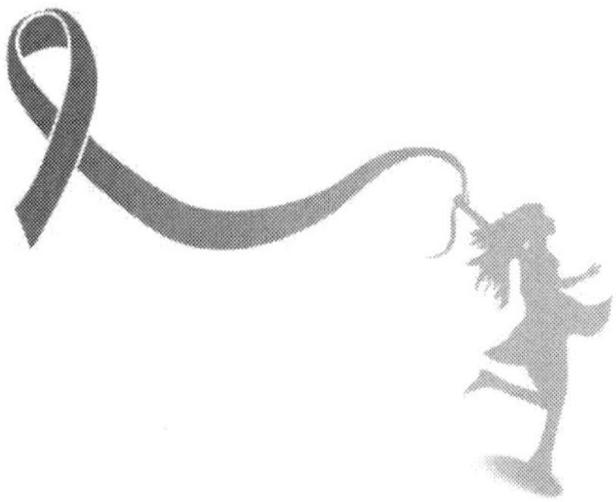

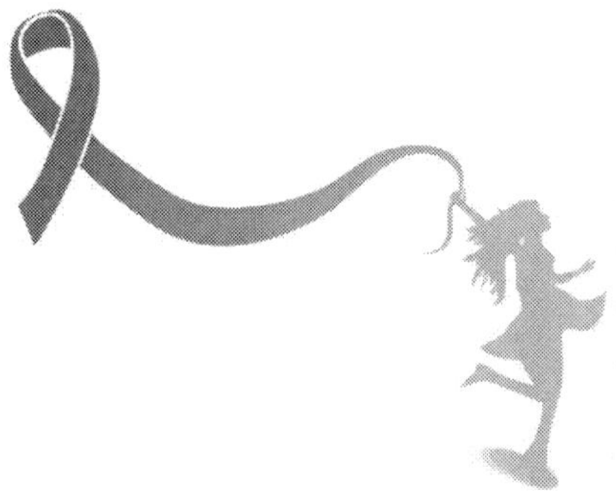

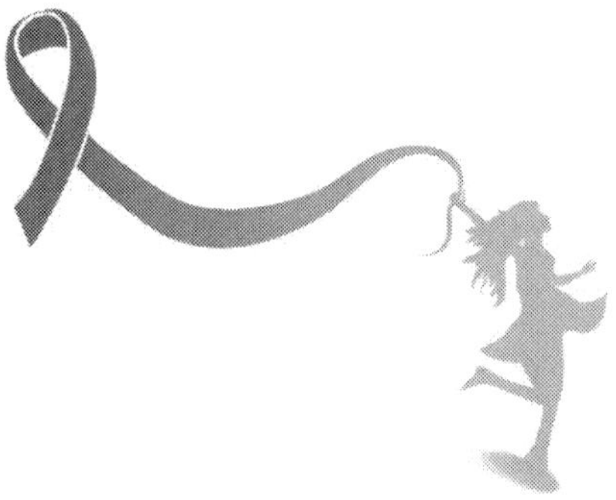

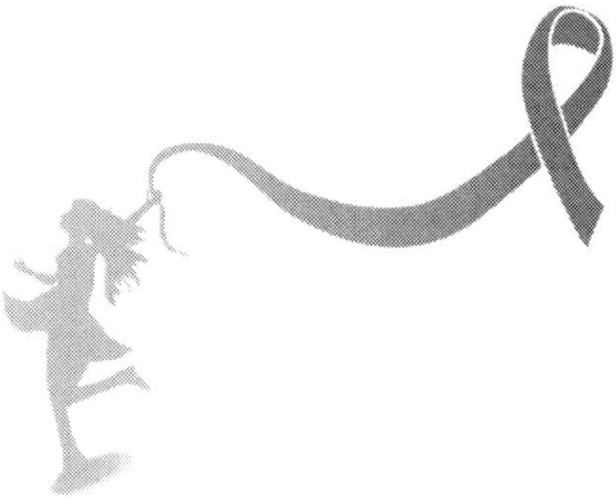

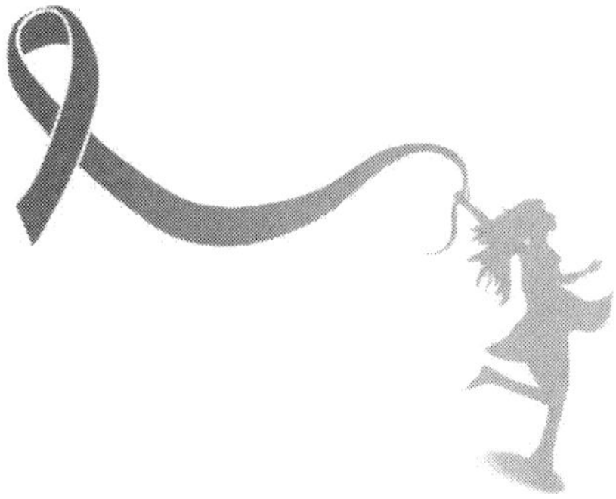

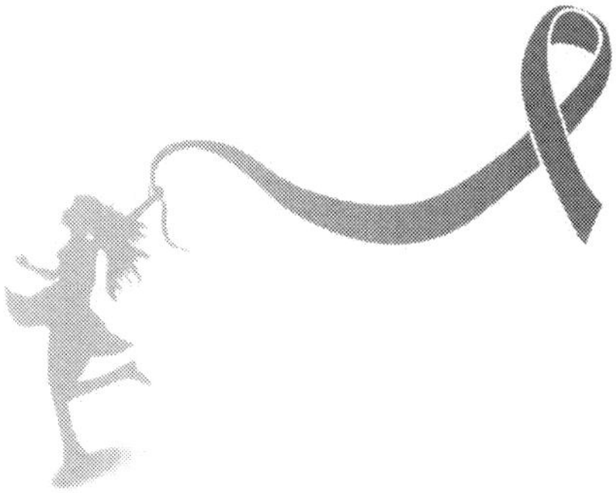

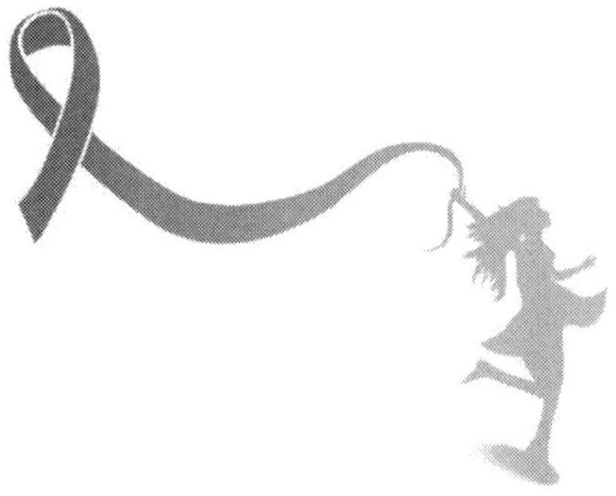

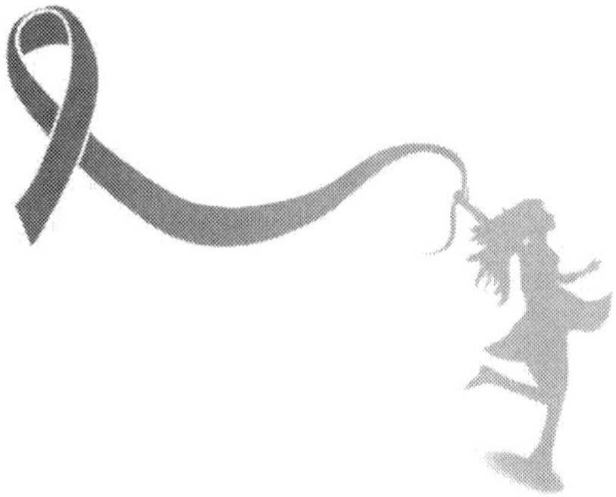

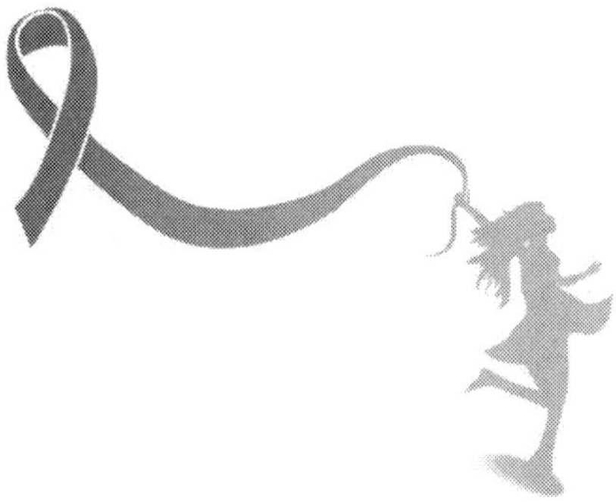

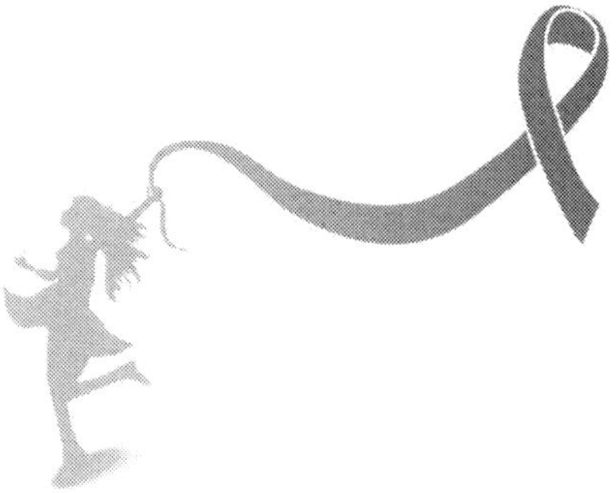

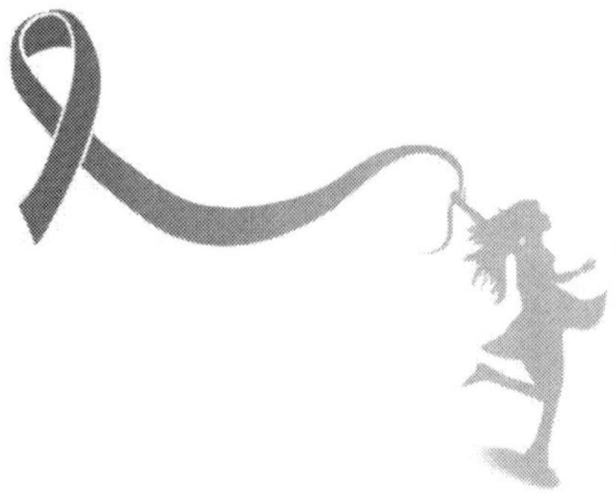

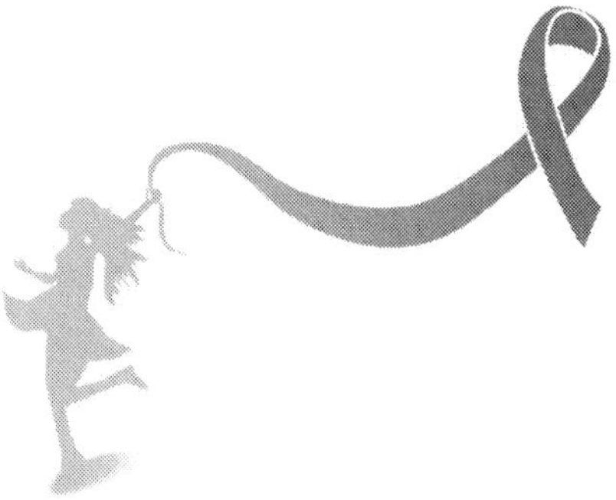

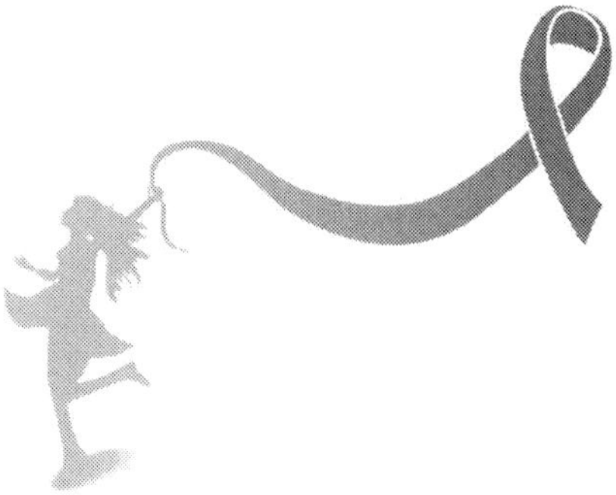

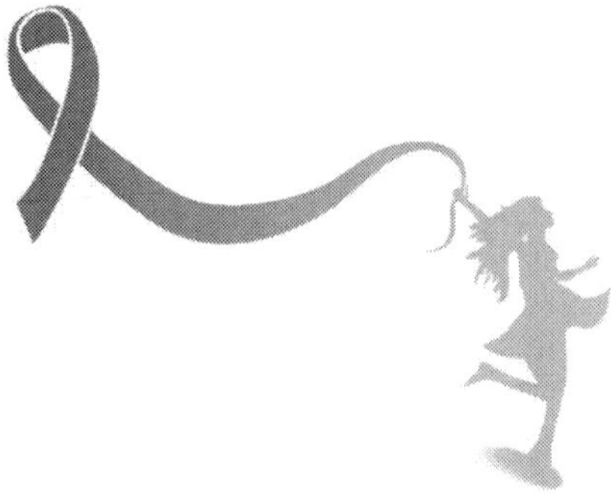

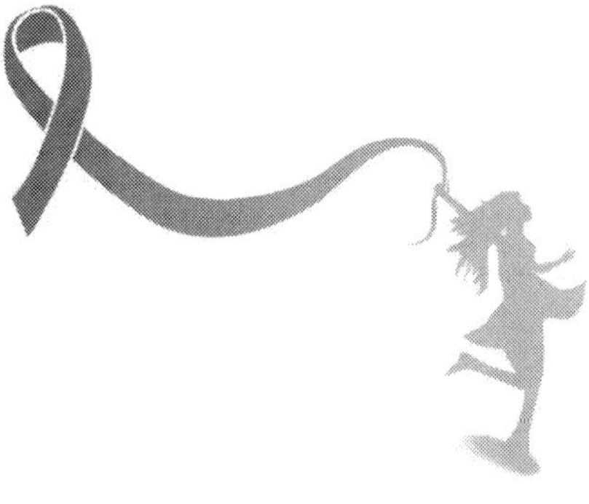

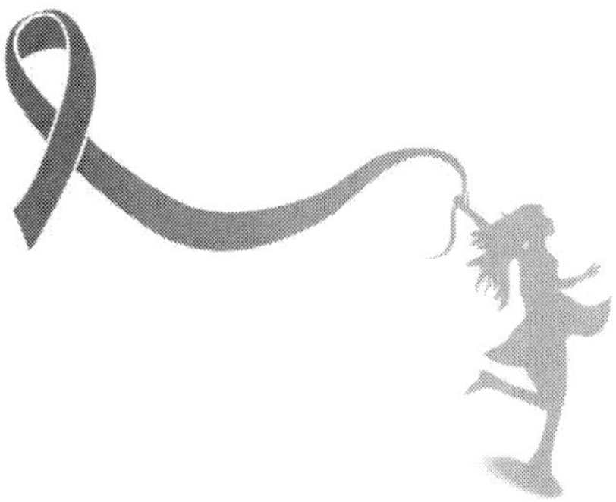

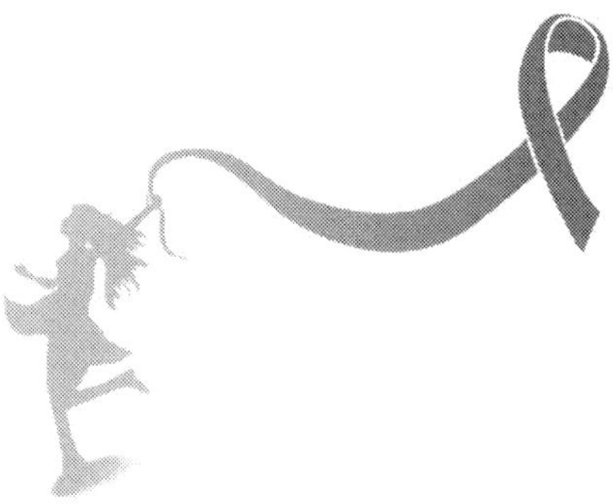

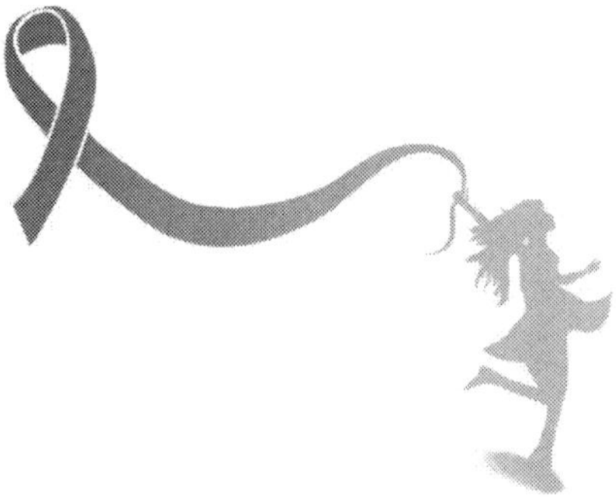

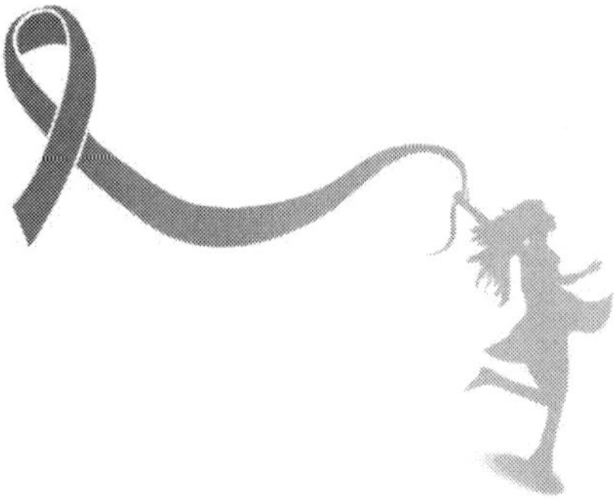

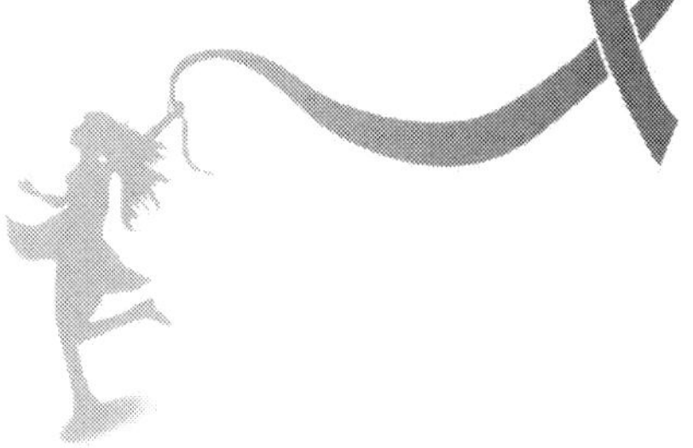

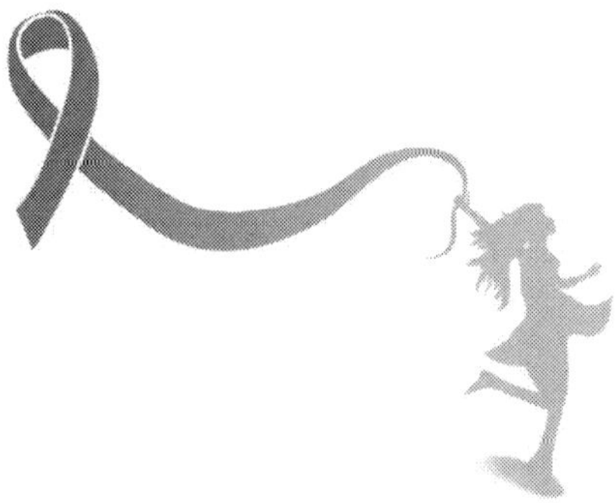

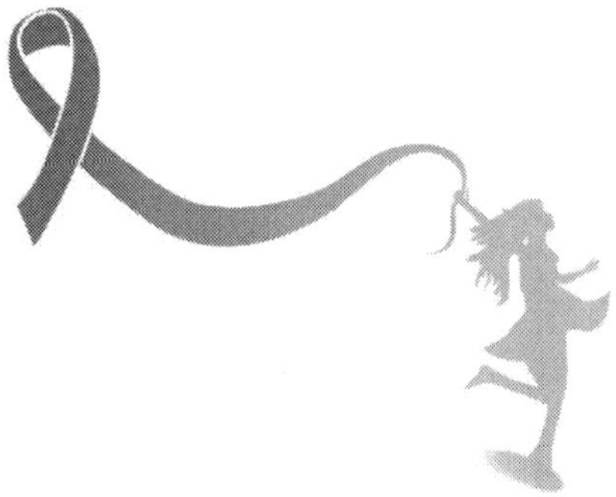

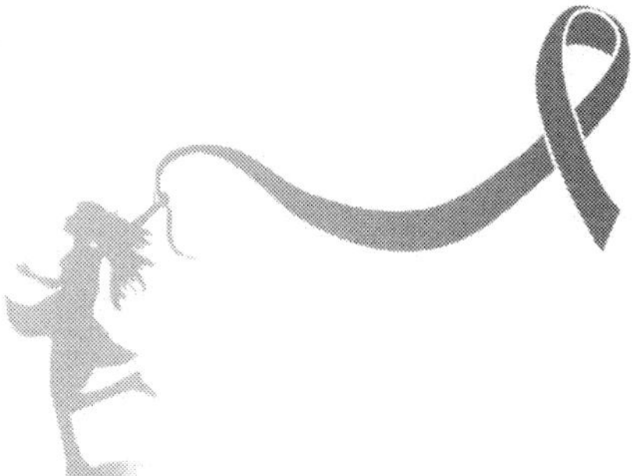

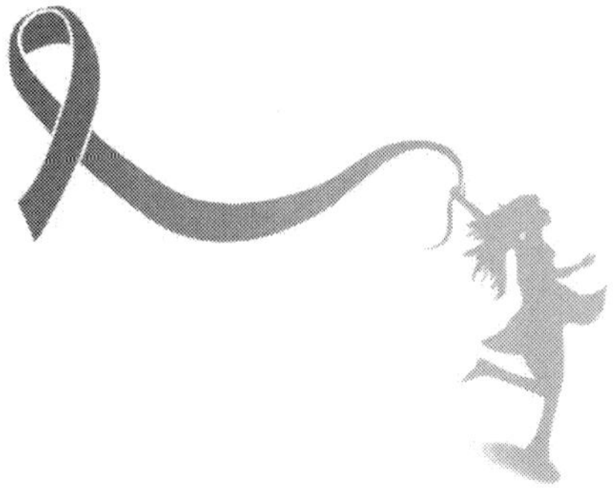

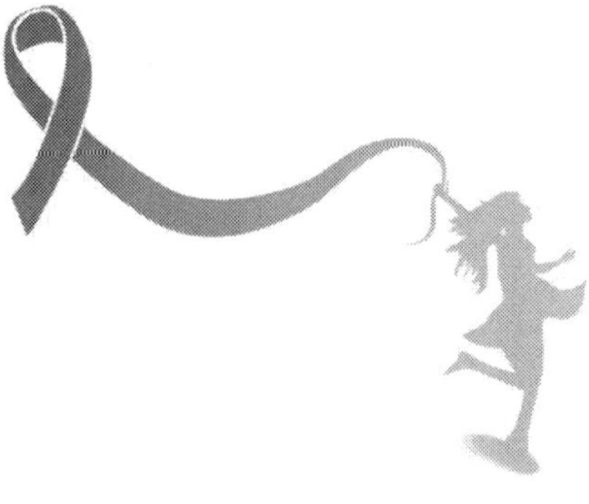

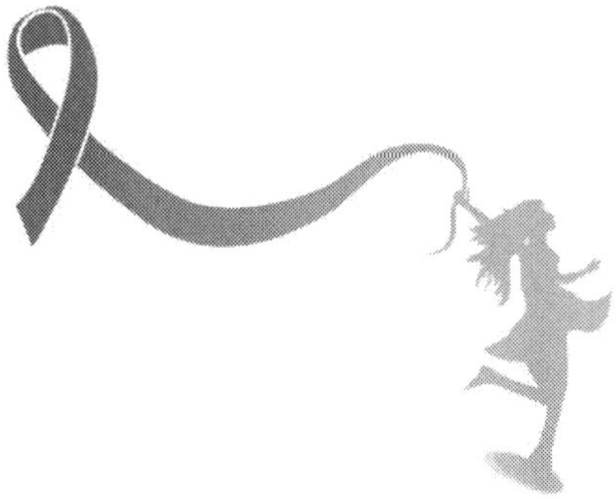

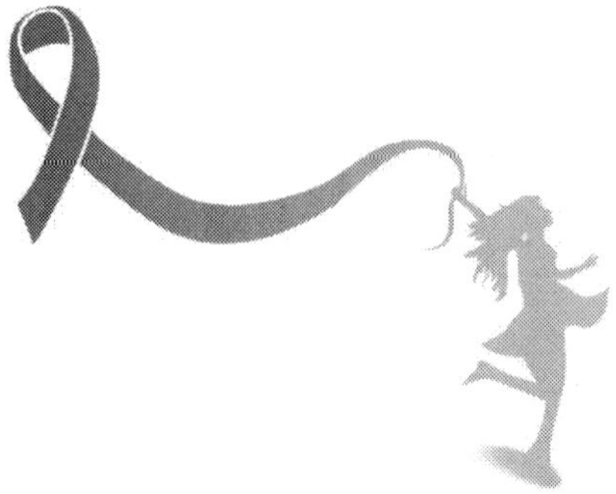

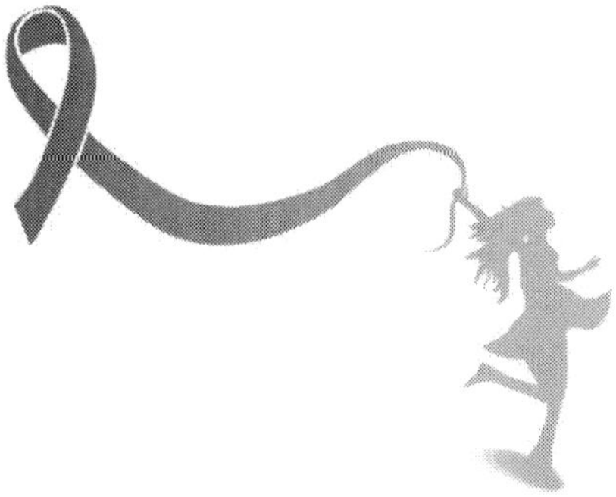

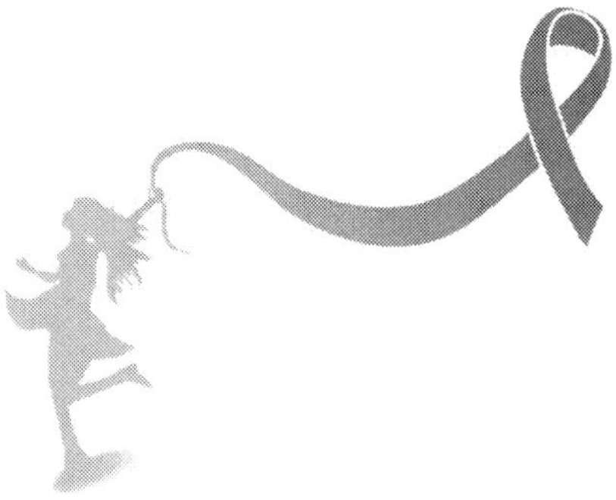

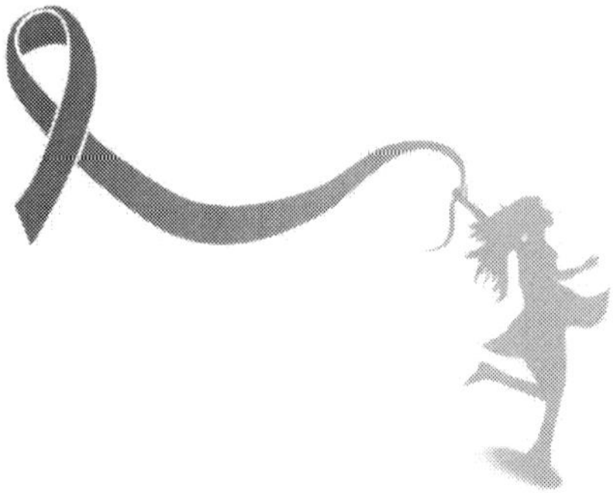

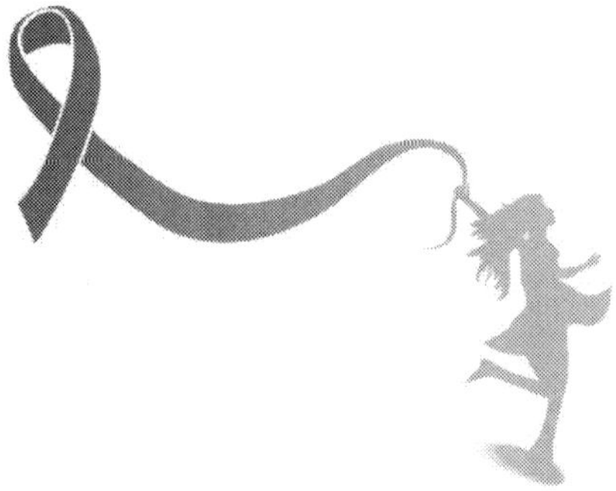

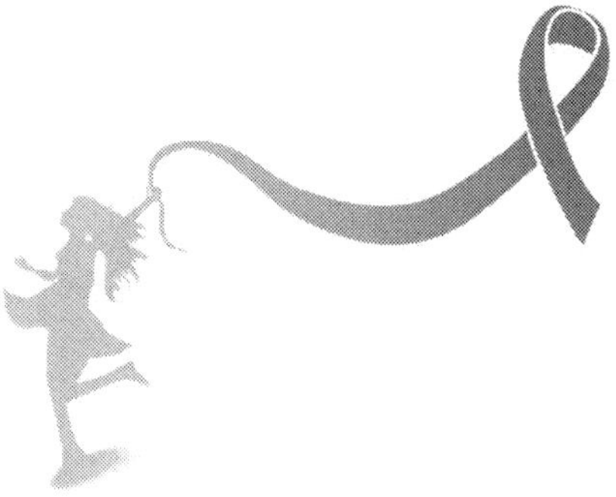

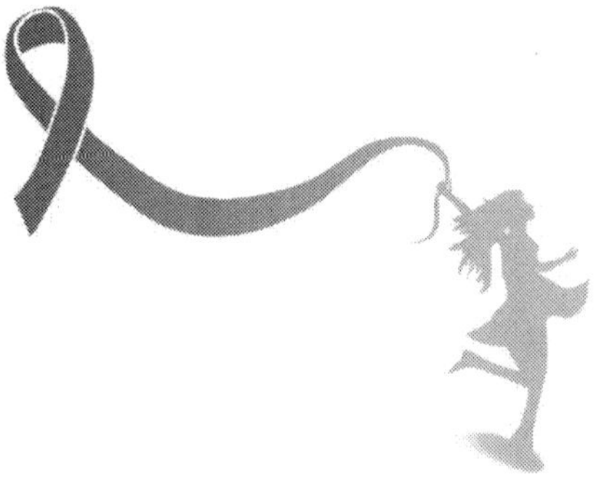

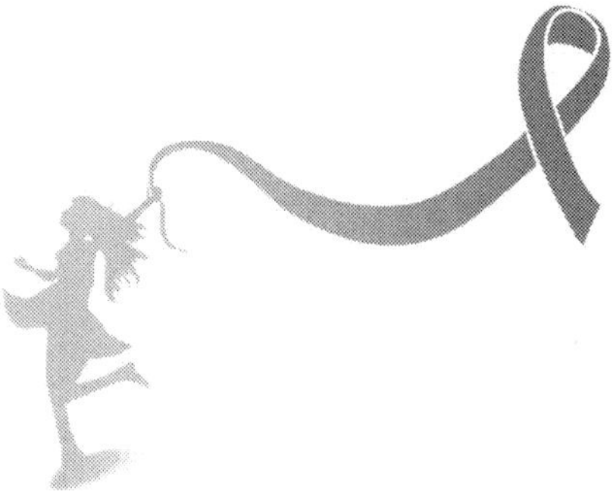

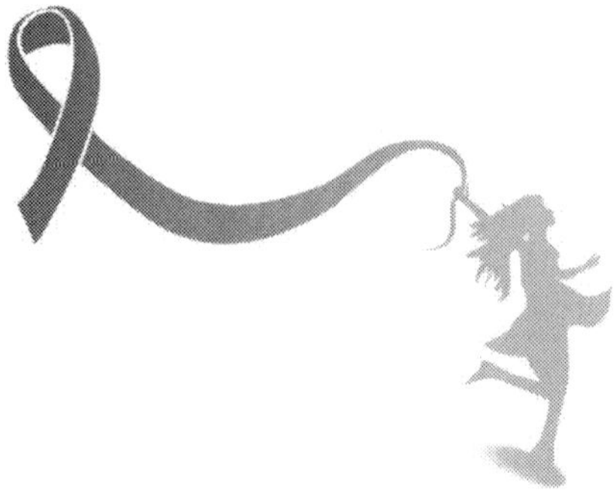

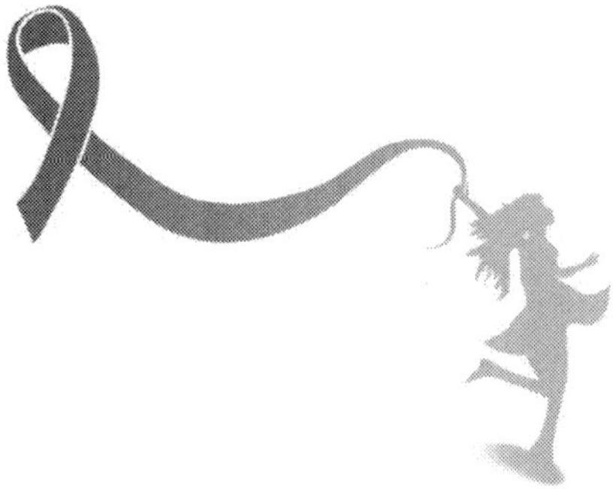

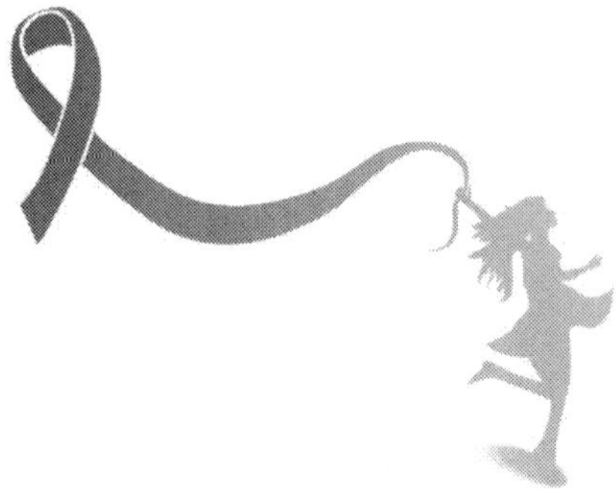

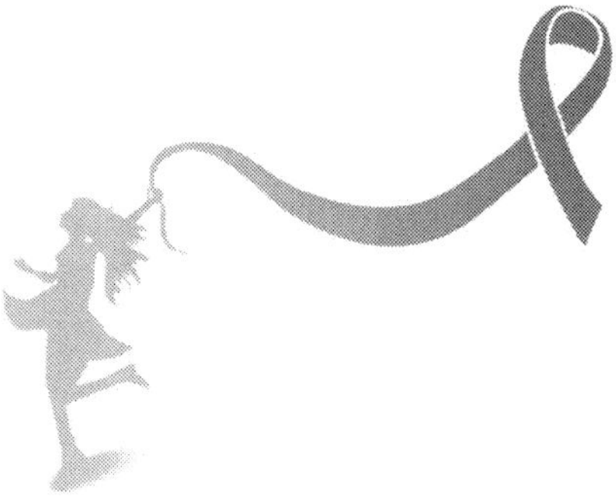

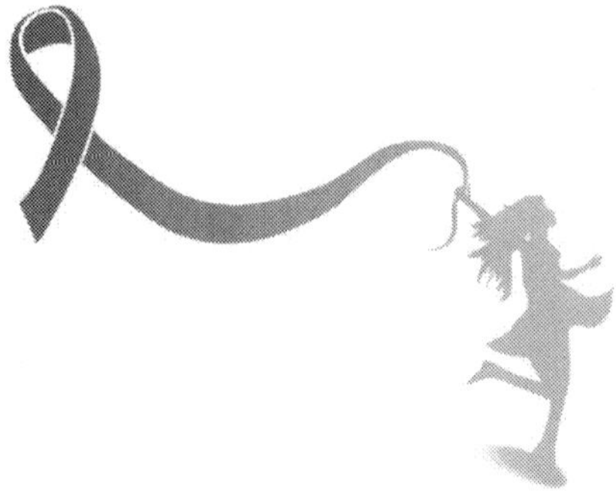

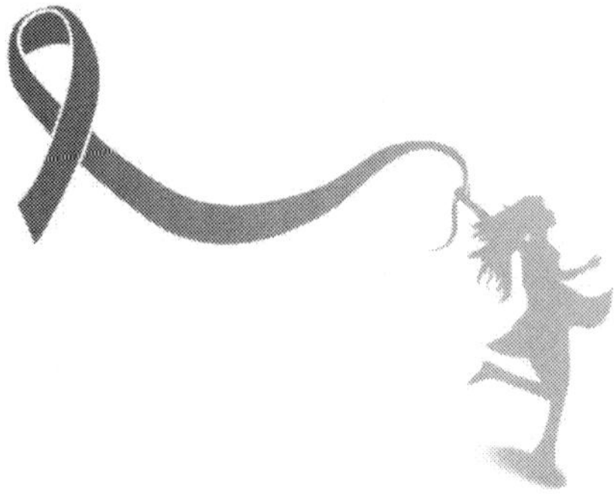

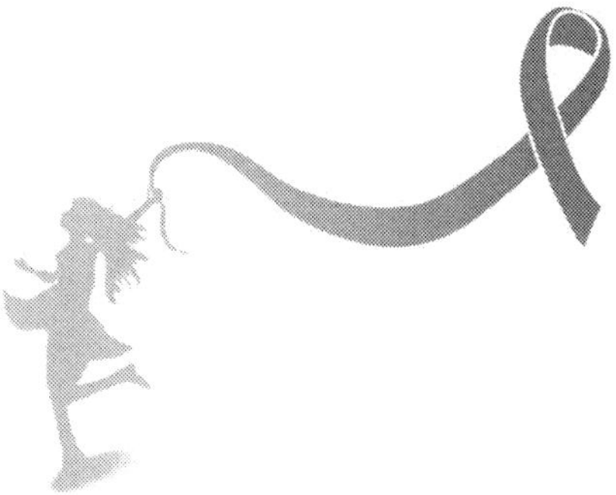

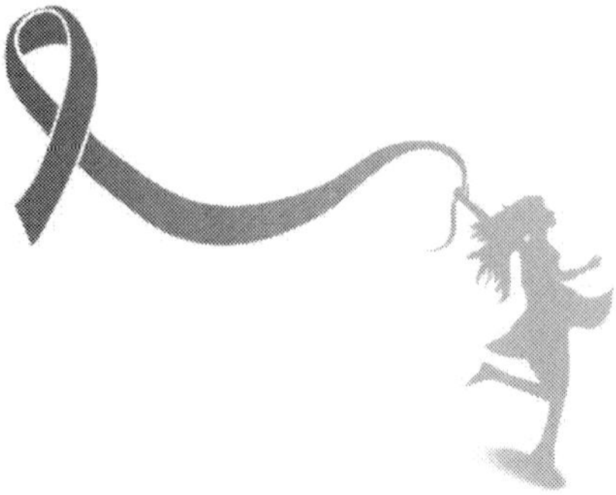

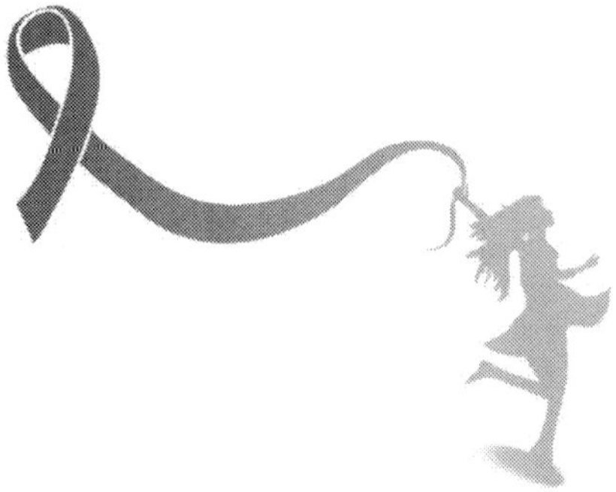

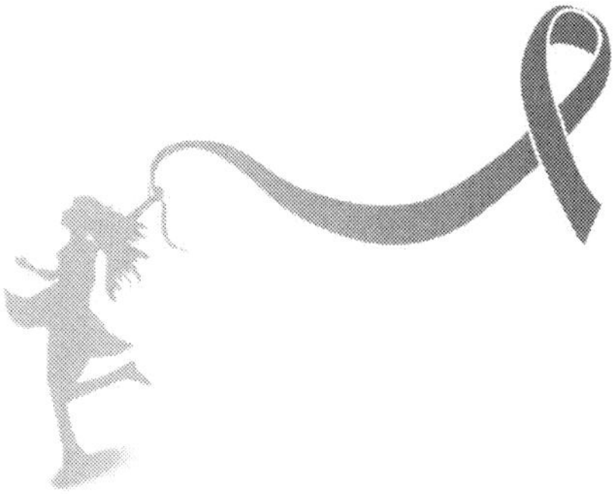

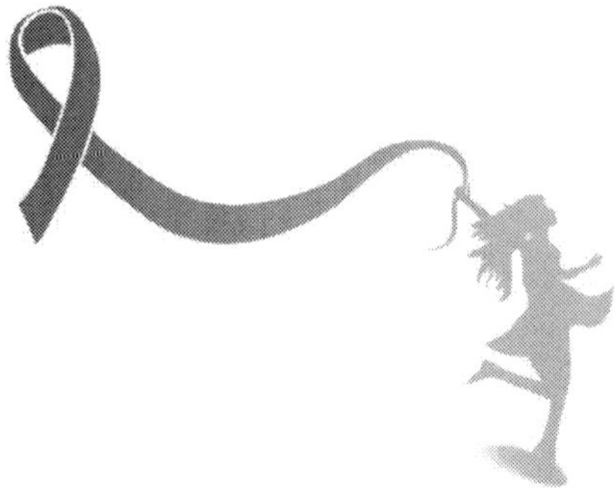

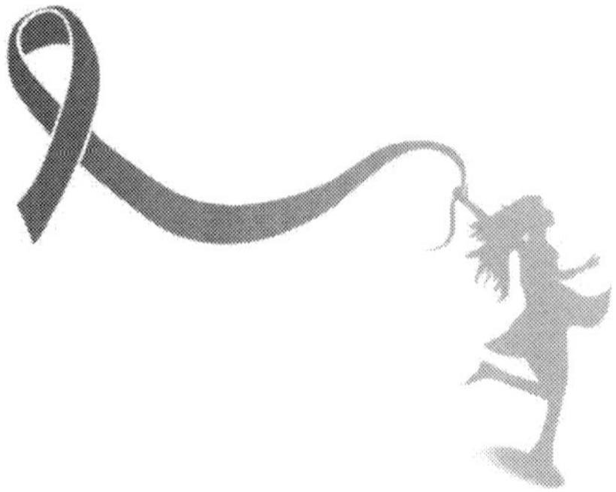

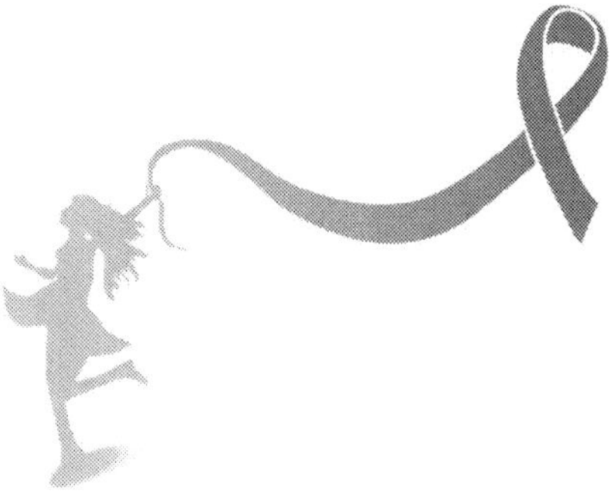

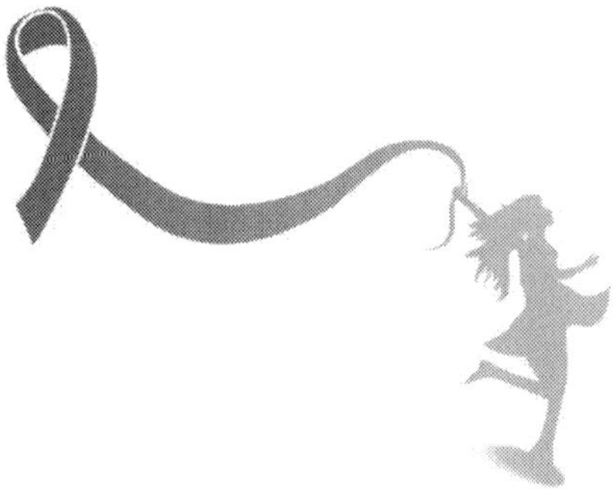

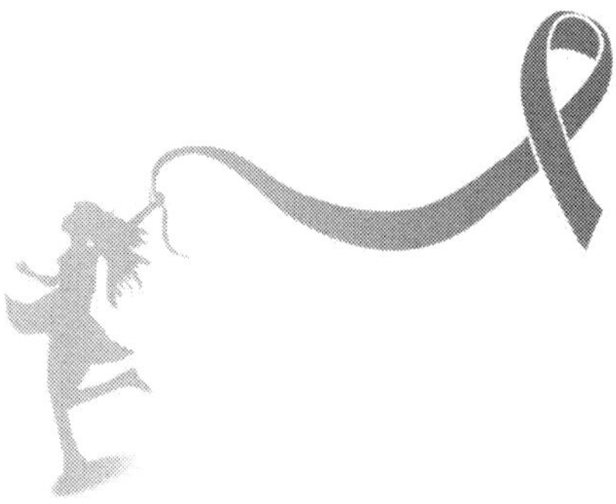

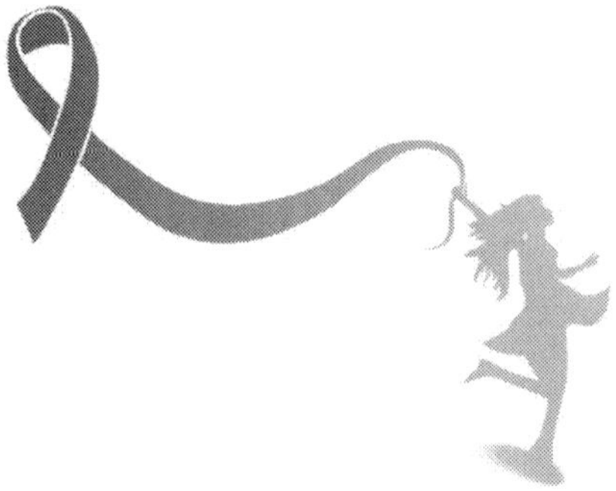

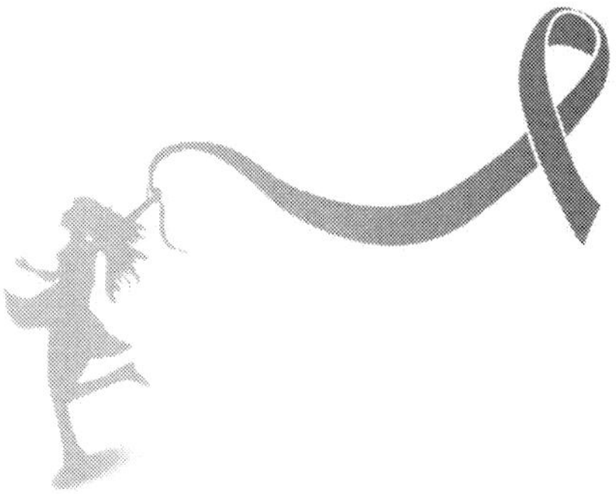

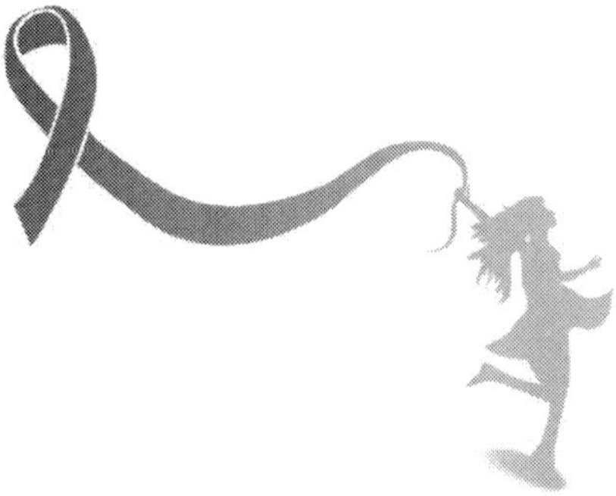

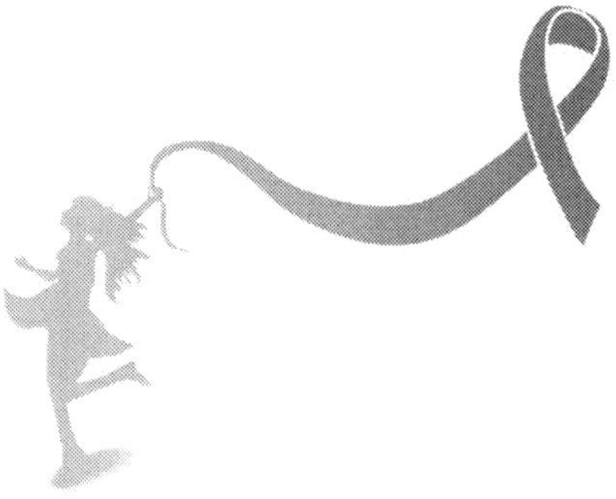

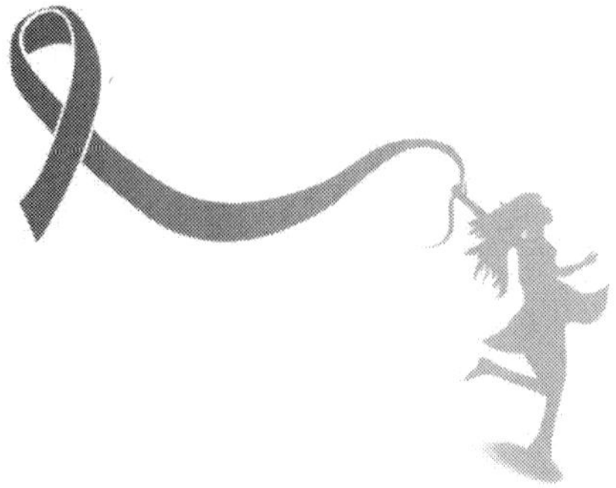

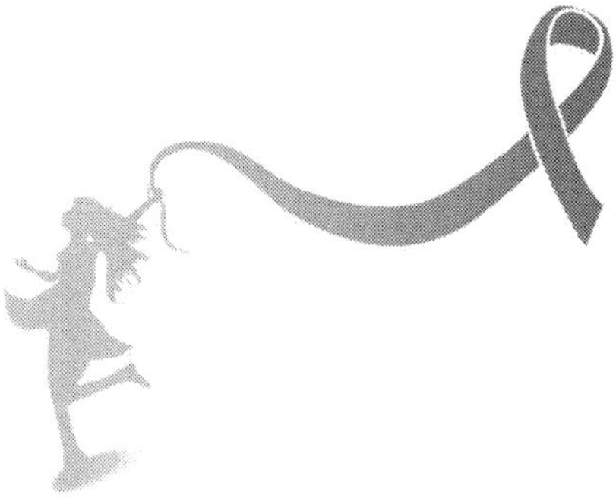

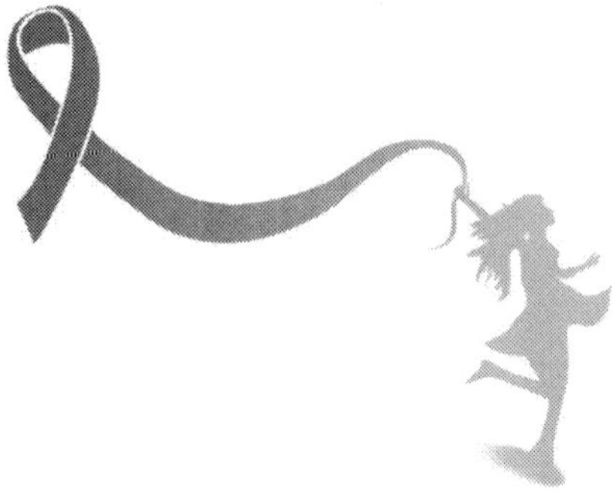

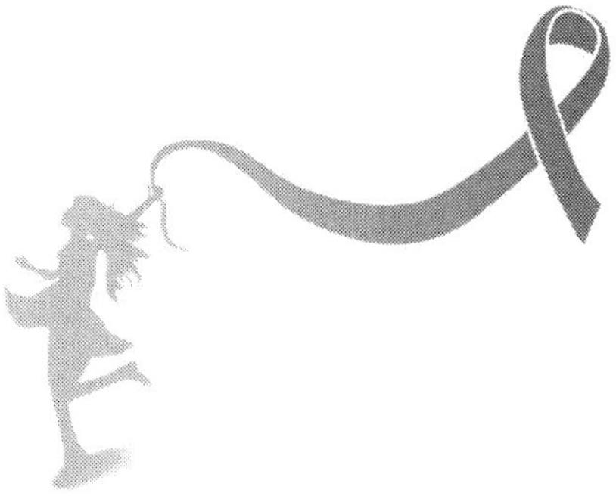

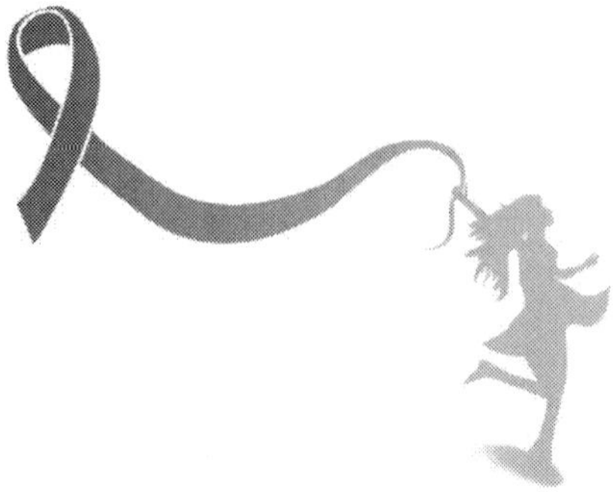

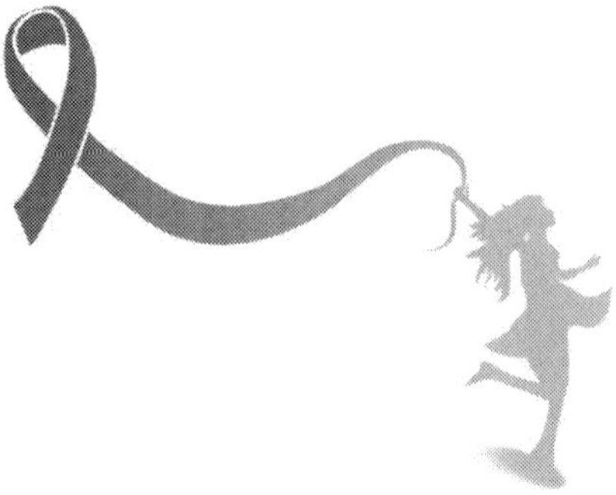

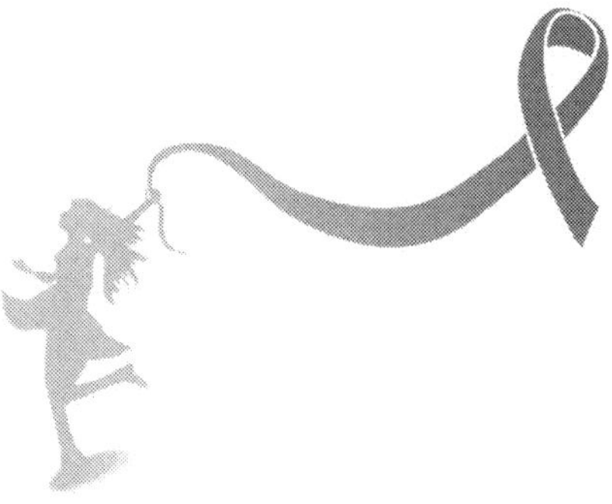

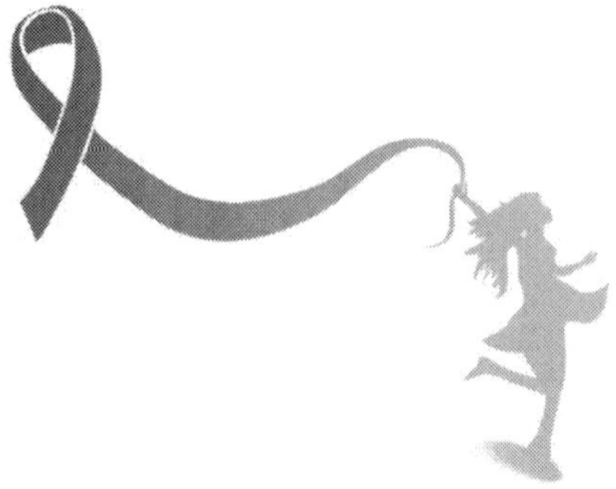

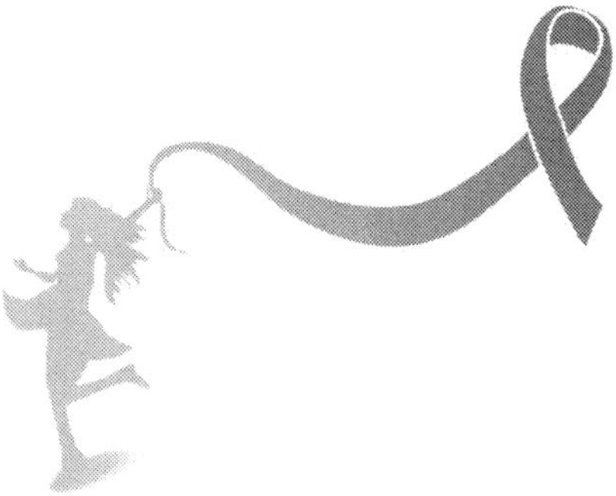

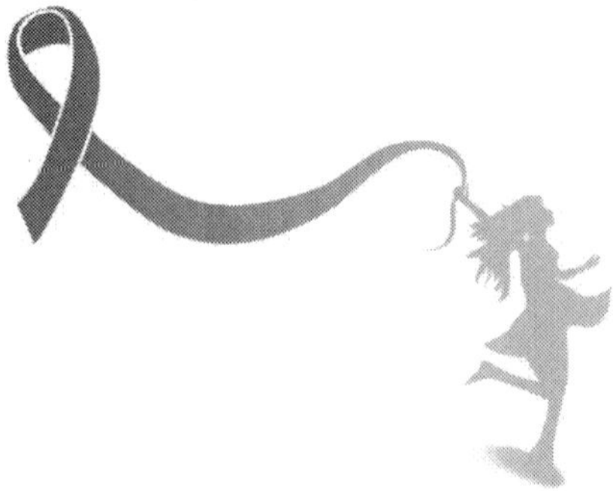

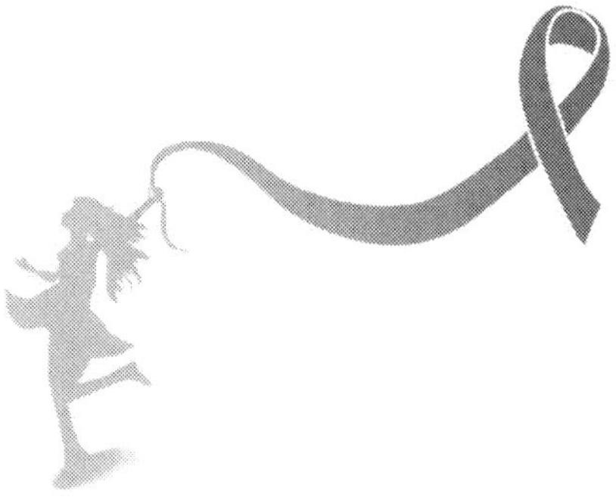

Made in the USA
Monee, IL
12 October 2021

79855306R10057